MW01148221

Building Bulk & Power
Revised Edition

Written and Published by Bill Pearl
Edited by George and Tuesday Coates
Layout and Illustrations by Richard R. Thornley Jr.

Copyright © 1963-2015 Bill Pearl

Bill Pearl
P.O. Box 1080
Phoenix, Oregon 97535
Email: support@billpearl.com
Website: www.billpearl.com

ISBN-13: 978-1-938855-10-8

Notice of Rights

All rights reserved. No part of this book may be reproduced or transmitted in any form by any means, electronic, mechanical, photocopying, recording, or otherwise, without the prior written permission of the publisher.

Medical Disclaimer - See Your Doctor

Most people may do all of the exercises found in this book with no ill effects. However, if certain movements cause discomfort they should be eliminated. See your doctor and get the doctor's approval on the total fitness program.

Table of Contents

Chapter 1

Introduction

Bulk is generally associated with Power. A big man is thought of as a strong man... IF he has the right kind of bodyweight!

The majority of men who exercise today are concerned with gaining bodyweight and/or strength. For those interested in Bulk and Power, here are three training programs personally used by Bill Pearl and Leo Stern and thousands of our students.

It may seem to you that the exercises in this book are very similar for each course. In a way this is true, but these exercises have been developed with but one goal in mind... Building Bulk and Power. What makes them effective is the way in which they are programmed. It is important that you follow these exercises exactly. Breathing is extremely important, as is the correct number of sets and repetitions. There is a definite relationship between these things... so do not improvise!

"We are born with faculties and powers capable of almost anything, such as at least would carry us further than can be easily imagined; but it is only the exercise of those powers which gives us ability and skill in anything, and leads us towards perfection."

John Locke

By using your God-given faculties and powers, you, too, can have bulk and power - size and strength. These courses are your guide. Use them wisely, for they are a proven road to perfection.

Good Luck!
Leo Stern

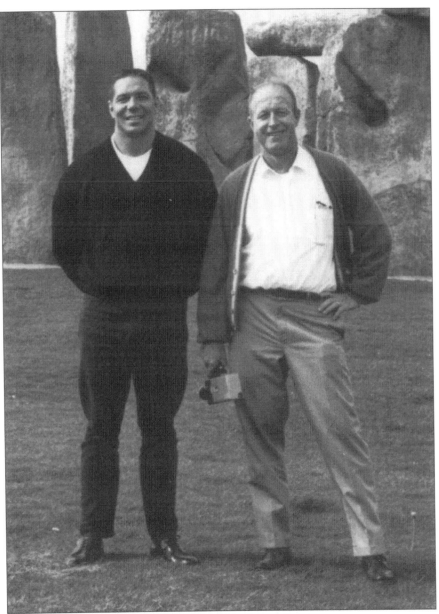

Bill and Leo Stern in 1961 with Stonehenge in the background.

Chapter 2

Building Bulk & Power

The major portion of this book is devoted to the training programs you should follow during your training period for Bulk and Power. We have outlined three scientifically planned programs for you to follow. It is recommended that you start with Course No. 1, regardless of how long you have trained. We agree that it may be less than what some of you are now doing in your training, but it will give your body a chance to rebuild itself and prepare your ligaments and tendons for the strain that will be placed on them in the two programs that follow.

All of the exercises are placed in the program exactly as they should be followed. In performing these exercises, it is important to do them exactly as prescribed in order to get a complete contraction and extension on each movement. At first, it is advisable to handle lighter weights in order to get the recommended repetitions. Do about two-thirds of your maximum effort on your exercises in the beginning. This will enable you to use a progressive method of adding weight to the exercises, as you follow the course.

While training for Bulk and Power, do not hurry through your sets; rest approximately 3-5 minutes between each set. This pace will enable you to use heavier weights as your stamina continues to build. Of course, your individual recuperative power will be the true measure of how fast a pace you should maintain. Because of the long rest periods between sets, we recommend you wear a sweat shirt. This will conserve energy that would normally be required to keep your body temperature to the point needed to get the maximum from your workout.

Keep accurate records of your training. Then, there will be no guesswork at your weights and sets and of your progress each week. Record your weight and be sure to weigh yourself before the workout and in the same training outfit each time. There is a fluctuation in everyone's bodyweight, so do not become discouraged if it bounces up and down from time to time. If you do not gain bodyweight in a period of a few weeks, you can then experiment by increasing your caloric intake and consuming more liquids. Do not expect a big increase in bodyweight the first week or two, for your system must adjust itself to the increased work.

Best of Luck,
Bill Pearl

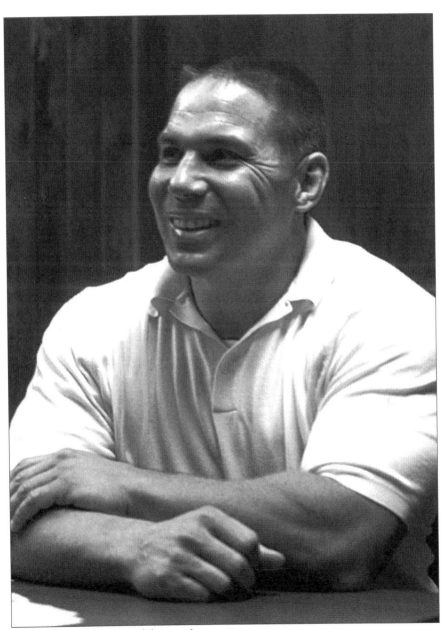

Bill Pearl smiling after a good days work.

Chapter 3

How to Use this Book

If a person is interested in weight training for more than basic conditioning, it is imperative that he study each illustration and description before attempting a new exercise. Progress definitely can be deterred if an exercise is done incorrectly.

Many exercises can be accomplished with the exact same motion but will affect different areas of a muscle by the angle at which the exercise is performed. For example: an exercise done on a flat bench, or an incline bench, will put different emphasis on the same muscle even though the same motion, weight and equipment are used.

It is therefore necessary to perform exercises from as many different angles that are reasonable and to use as many variations that are reasonable to develop a fully matured muscular physique.

On the following pages, highly accurate drawings appear that will enable you to see the pieces of equipment used to perform each exercise and the style used for each movement. Each exercise includes the proper name of the exercise, the muscle group most affected, "degree of difficulty" information, and a written description of how the exercise should be done.

The "degree of difficulty" information appearing below each exercise heading will give you at a glance what exercise may be suited for your present physical condition.

NOTE: It is not necessarily true that an exercise considered "easy" may not be just as effective as one considered "hard". Any exercise can be made more or less difficult, depending on the weight used or the effort put forth.

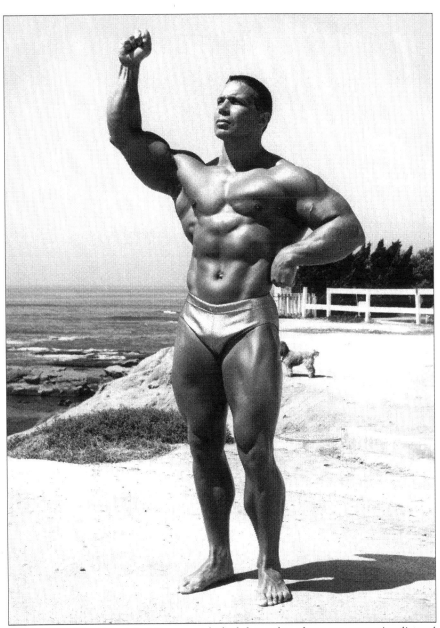

At this stage of Pearl's bodybuilding career, he had changed to a lacto-ovo-vegetarian diet and was still able to maintain his massive size and strength.

Chapter 4

Equipment Needed

Equipment needed to perform the exercises in this training guide.

- Barbell
- Dumbbells
- Flat Bench
- Incline Bench
- Stool
- Block
- Abdominal Board

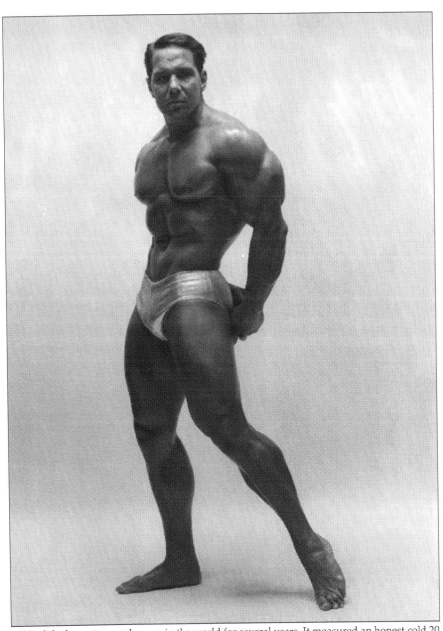

Bill had the largest muscular arm in the world for several years. It measured an honest cold 20 3/8 inches at a bodyweight of 218 pounds.

Chapter 5

Course One

EXERCISES:

1. Warm Up (Dumbbell Swing Through)	1 set of 10
2. Flat Bench Twisting Leg Raise	1 set of 30
3. Barbell Good Morning	1 set of 10
4. Flat Footed Wide Stance Barbell Squat	2 sets of 15
5. Bent Arm Lateral	2 sets of 12
6. Standing Barbell Toe Raise	3 sets of 20
7. Barbell Shoulder Shrug	2 sets of 8
8. Medium Grip Barbell Bench Press	2 sets of 8
9. Medium Grip Bent Over Barbell Rowing	2 sets of 8
10. Standing Military Press	2 sets of 8
11. Standing Medium Grip Barbell Curl	2 sets of 8
12. Barbell Dead Lift	3 sets of 5

- Follow this course of exercises for a six weeks period
- Do Three Workouts per Week
- Note alternate exercises 4 and 5

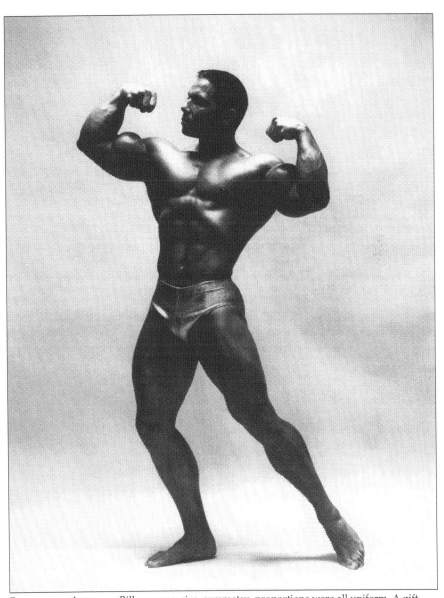

From any angle or pose Bill assumes, size, symmetry, proportions were all uniform. A gift from God and hard work.

WARM-UP (DUMBBELL SWING-THROUGH)

Muscle Group: Most large muscle groups
Degree of Difficulty: Easy

Grasp a dumbbell with both hands. Stand erect with your feet about sixteen inches apart. With your arms straight, bend at the waist until your upper back is parallel with the floor. Inhale and raise up with the dumbbell held at arm's length until it is directly overhead as you come to an erect position. Lower the dumbbell back to starting position in the same semicircular motion you raised it and exhale. Try to swing the dumbbell through your legs to stretch as much as possible before repeating the next repetition.

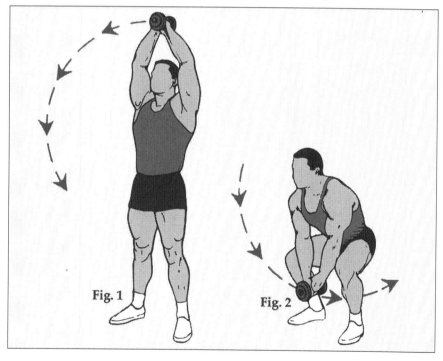

Fig. 1   Fig. 2

FLAT BENCH TWISTING LEG RAISE

Muscle Group: Lower abdominals and obliques
Degree of Difficulty: Intermediate

Lie on a flat bench with your legs off the end of the bench. Place your hands under your buttocks with your palms facing down. With your legs locked out, twist your hips slightly to the right. Inhale and raise your legs until they are vertical above your hips. Lower your legs until they are about three inches off the floor and exhale. Do the prescribed number of repetitions on the right side and then change the angle of your hips to the left side and repeat the same number of repetitions.

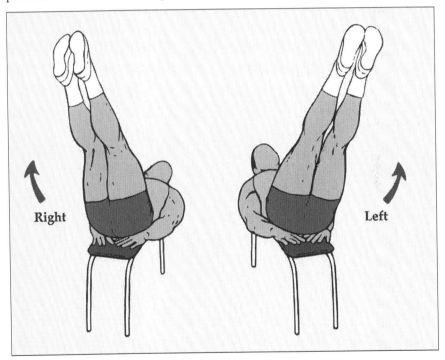

Right   Left

BARBELL GOOD MORNING

Muscle Group: Lower back and abdominals
Degree of Difficulty: Easy

Stand erect with your feet about sixteen inches apart. Place a light barbell on your shoulders. Grasp the bar with both hands in a comfortable position. Keep your back straight and your head up as you inhale and bend forward at the waist until your upper body is parallel to the floor. Return to starting position and exhale. Be sure your knees are in a locked position during the entire exercise.

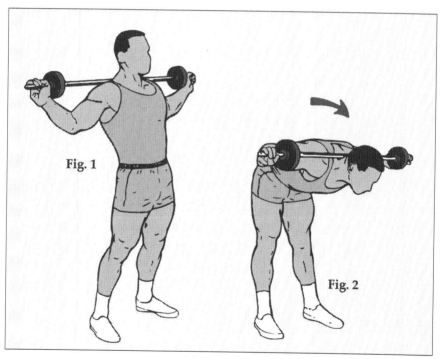

Fig. 1

Fig. 2

FLAT FOOTED WIDE STANCE BARBELL SQUAT TO BENCH

Muscle Group: Inner thighs
Degree of Difficulty: Intermediate

Place a bench that is about sixteen inches high behind you and stand close enough to the bench so your heels are about even with the end of the bench closest to you. Place a barbell on your upper back. Help stabilize the bar with a hand grip and spacing that feels most comfortable to you. Keep your head up, back straight, and your feet planted firmly on the floor about thirty inches apart. Inhale and squat down until your buttocks touch the bench. Do not take the tension off your thighs and totally sit on the bench. Your head should remain up, back straight, and your knees pointing outward. Return to starting position and exhale.

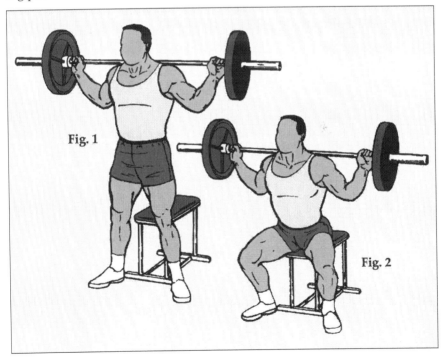

Fig. 1

Fig. 2

BENT ARM LATERAL

Muscle Group: Outer pectorals
Degree of Difficulty: Intermediate

Lie on a flat bench with the dumbbells together at arm's length above the shoulders The palms of the hands should be facing each other. Slowly lower the dumbbells to the down position so the dumbbells are approximately even with the chest but out about ten inches from each side of the chest. Notice that the elbows are drawn downwards and back so they are in line with the ears. The forearms are slightly out of a vertical position. The press back to starting position is done by using the same arc as in letting the dumbbells down. Inhale at the beginning of the exercise and exhale at the finish.

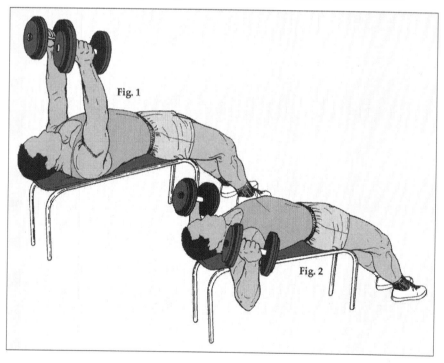

Fig. 1

Fig. 2

STANDING BARBELL TOE RAISE

Muscle Group: Main calf muscles
Degree of Difficulty: Intermediate

Place a barbell on the back of your shoulders. Step on a thick board or raised platform. Place your feet on the raised object to help balance yourself and to get a full extension and contraction of the calf muscle. Place your heels down. Inhale and push up on your toes as shown in illustration #1. This position is the flexed portion of the exercise and the lowering of the heels is the extension portion. Both are important. Do the exercise slowly and deliberately. Inhale as you raise on your toes and exhale as you lower your heels. If you turn your toes out and heels in, it will affect the inner calf more. If you keep your feet straight, it will affect the main calf muscle more. If you turn your toes in and heels out, it will affect the outside of the calf more.

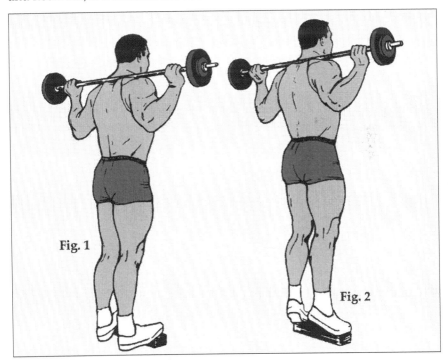

Fig. 1
Fig. 2

BARBELL SHOULDER SHRUG

Muscle Group: Trapezius
Degree of Difficulty: Intermediate

Place a barbell on the floor in front of you. With a foot stance about sixteen inches apart, bend down and grasp the bar with both hands about twenty-four inches apart. Stand erect with the bar hanging in front of you at arm's length. Drop both shoulders down to the front of you as much as possible. Inhale and raise your shoulders up and rotate them in a circular motion from the front to the rear returning to the starting position at the end of the repetition. Exhale as you return to starting position. Keep your back straight.

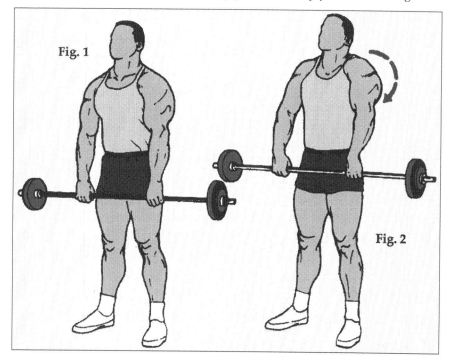

Fig. 1

Fig. 2

MEDIUM GRIP BARBELL BENCH PRESS

Muscle Group: Outer pectorals
Degree of Difficulty: Intermediate

Lie in a supine position on a flat bench with your legs positioned at the sides of the bench and your feet flat on the floor. Using a hand grip that is about six inches wider than your shoulder width, bring the barbell to arm's length above the chest but in line with the shoulders. Lower the barbell to a position on the chest that is about an inch below the nipples of the pectorals. Note from the illustration that the elbows are back and the chest is held high. Inhale as the barbell is lowered to the chest and exhale as you push the barbell back to arm's length. Do not relax and drop the weight on the chest but lower it with complete control making a definite pause at the chest before pressing it back to starting position. Keep the head on the bench and do not arch the back too sharply as to raise your hips off the bench.

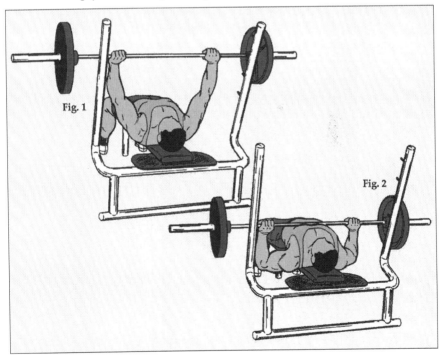

Fig. 1

Fig. 2

MEDIUM GRIP BENT OVER BARBELL ROWING

Muscle Group: Lats
Degree of Difficulty: Intermediate

Place a barbell on the floor in front of you. With your feet about eighteen inches apart bend down and get a grip on the barbell that is about twenty-six inches wide. Keep the legs bent and your back parallel to the floor as you inhale and pull the barbell directly up to the lower part of your chest. Exhale as the barbell returns to starting position. Do not let the barbell touch the floor once you have begun the exercise. Keep your head up and your back straight.

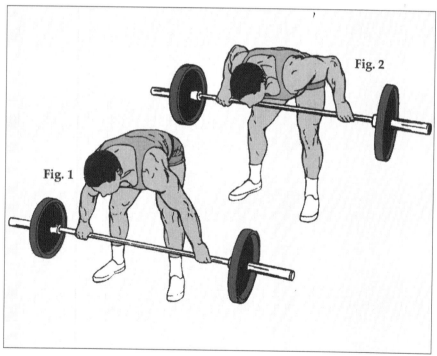

Fig. 2

Fig. 1

STANDING MILITARY PRESS

Muscle Group: Front and outer deltoids
Degree of Difficulty: Intermediate

This is the standard military press. Clean the weight to the chest. Lock the legs and hips solidly. This will give you a solid platform from which to push. Keep the elbows in slightly and under the bar, press the weight overhead, lock the arms out. When lowering the barbell to the upper chest, be sure it rests on the chest and is not held with the arms. If the chest is held high, it will give you a nice shelf on which to place the barbell and to push from. Inhale before the press and exhale when lowering the barbell.

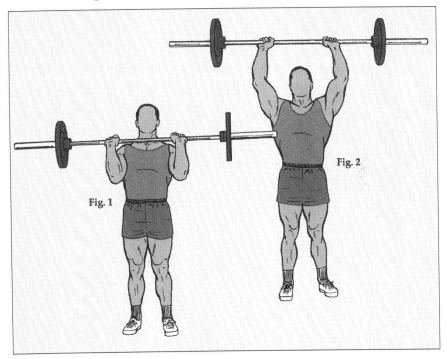

Fig. 1

Fig. 2

STANDING MEDIUM GRIP BARBELL CURL

Muscle Group: Biceps
Degree of Difficulty: Intermediate

Hold a barbell with both hands using a palms-up grip about eighteen inches apart. Stand erect with your feet about sixteen inches apart. With the barbell at arm's length against your upper thighs, inhale and curl the bar up to the height of your shoulders keeping your back straight, legs and hips locked out. As you are lowering the bar back to starting position, do so in a controlled manner causing the biceps to resist the weight as much as possible. Exhale as you return to starting position.

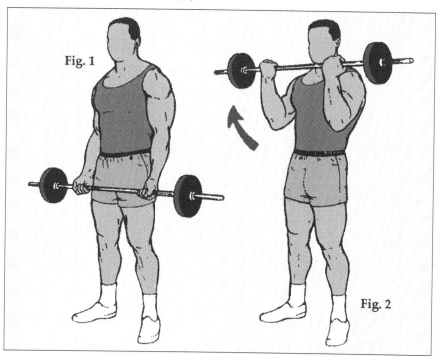

Fig. 1

Fig. 2

BARBELL DEAD LIFT

Muscle Group: Lower back
Degree of Difficulty: Intermediate

Place a barbell on the floor in front of you. With your feet about sixteen inches apart, bend down and grasp the bar just to the outside of your knees in the middle of your lower legs. Keep your knees bent and your back straight while you have your head up. Inhale and, using your thighs and back, stand erect with your arms locked out. Lower the weight to the floor and exhale.

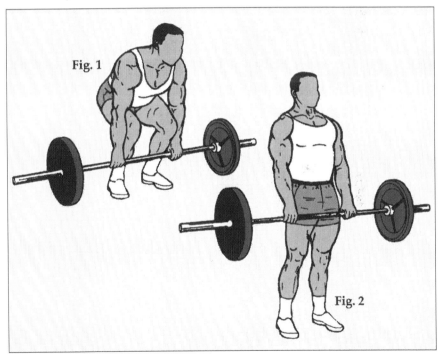

Fig. 1

Fig. 2

Chapter 6

Course Two

EXERCISES:

1. Warm-Up (Dumbbell Swing-Through)	1 set of 10-15
2. Bent Knee Sit-Up	1 set of 15-50
3. Dumbbell Side Bend	1 set of 15-50
4. Seated Flat Bench Leg Pull-In	1 set of 10-30
5. Flat Footed Wide Stance Barbell Squat	3-5 sets of 6-8
6. Bent Arm Barbell Pullover	3-5 sets of 8-10
7. Standing Barbell Toe Raise	3 sets of 15-20
8. Medium Grip Barbell Upright Rowing	2 sets of 8
9. Standing Military Press	2 sets of 5-6
10. Hand on Bench One Arm Dumbbell Rowing	3 sets of 8
11. Barbell Dead Lift	2 sets of 8
12. Incline Lateral	2 sets of 6-8
13. Bent Arm Lateral	2 sets of 6-8
14. Standing Dumbbell Triceps Curl	3 sets of 6-8
15. Standing Dumbbell Curl	3 sets of 6-8

- Follow this course of exercises for a six weeks period
- Do Three Workouts per Week

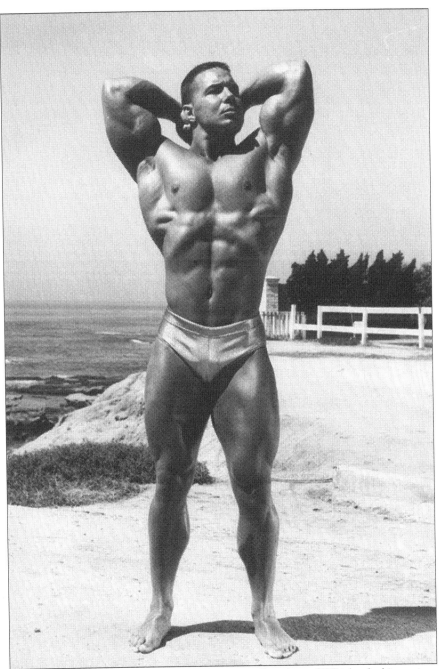

Bulk, power, and symmetry personified in this outstanding photo of Bill taken by his mentor Leo Stern.

WARM-UP (DUMBBELL SWING-THROUGH)

Muscle Group: Most large muscle groups
Degree of Difficulty: Easy

Grasp a dumbbell with both hands. Stand erect with your feet about sixteen inches apart. With your arms straight, bend at the waist until your upper back is parallel with the floor. Inhale and raise up with the dumbbell held at arm's length until it is directly overhead as you come to an erect position. Lower the dumbbell back to starting position in the same semicircular motion you raised it and exhale. Try to swing the dumbbell through your legs to stretch as much as possible before repeating the next repetition.

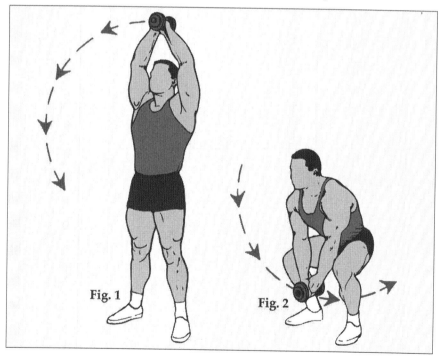

Fig. 1   Fig. 2

BENT KNEE SIT-UP

Muscle Group: Upper abdominals
Degree of Difficulty: Intermediate

Sit down on a sit-up board and hook your feet under the strap. With your knees bent to about a 45° angle, put your hands behind your head and place your chin on your chest. This will keep a slight bow to your back. From this position, inhale and lie back until your lower back touches the board. Exhale as you return to starting position.

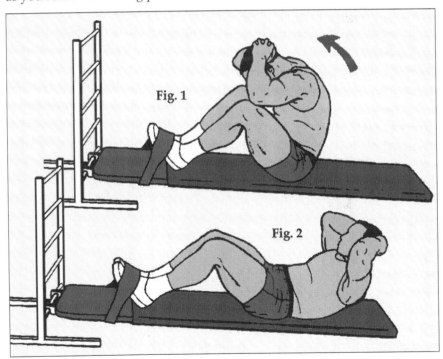

Fig. 1

Fig. 2

DUMBBELL SIDE BEND

Muscle Group: Obliques
Degree of Difficulty: Intermediate

Stand erect with your feet about sixteen inches apart and grasp a dumbbell in your right hand. Your palm will be facing your upper thigh. Place your left hand on your left oblique. Inhale and bend to the right as far as possible and then bend to the left as far as possible and exhale. You will perform the prescribed number of repetitions and then change the weight to the left hand and repeat the movement. You must remember to keep your back straight and your head up or you will bend too far forward.

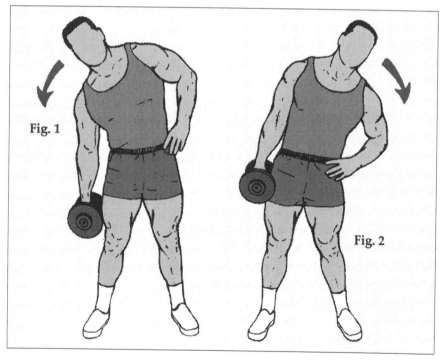

Fig. 1

Fig. 2

SEATED FLAT BENCH LEG PULL-IN

Muscle Group: Lower abdominals
Degree of Difficulty: Intermediate

Sit down on the end of a flat bench with your legs straight out in front of you. Place your hands behind your buttocks and grasp the outer sides of the bench for support. Inhale and bend your knees while pulling your upper thighs into your midsection. Return to starting position and exhale. Concentrate on your abdominals during the exercise. Note that your lower legs are parallel to the floor at the halfway point of the exercise.

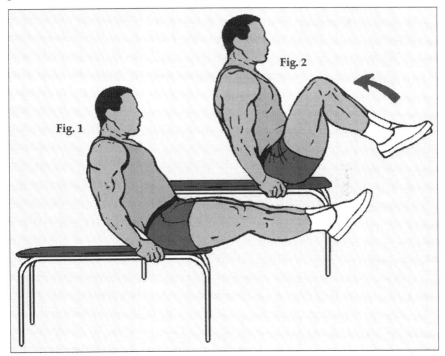

Fig. 1

Fig. 2

FLAT FOOTED WIDE STANCE BARBELL SQUAT

Muscle Group: Inner thighs
Degree of Difficulty: Intermediate

Place a barbell on your upper back. Help stabilize the bar with a hand grip and spacing that feels most comfortable to you. Keep your head up, back straight, and your feet planted firmly on the floor about thirty inches apart. Inhale and squat down until your upper thighs are parallel with the floor. Your head should remain up, back straight, and knees pointing outward. Return to starting position and exhale.

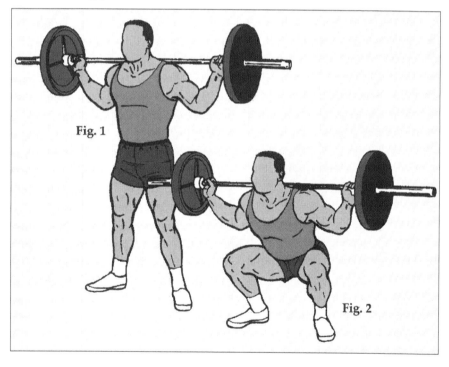

Fig. 1

Fig. 2

BENT ARM BARBELL PULLOVER

Muscle Group: Upper pectorals and rib cage
Degree of Difficulty: Intermediate

Lie supine on a flat bench with your shoulders at the end of the bench and your head pointing downward towards the floor. With a barbell on your chest resting in line with the nipples of the pectorals, use a hand grip that is about fourteen inches wide. Keeping the elbows in during the entire exercise, take a deep breath and lower the weight over your chest and face, keeping the barbell as close to the body as you can without scraping your nose. Continue to lower the weight until it touches the floor, or as low as is a comfortable position for you. Pull the barbell back to the chest, using the same path in which you lowered it. Exhale as you are doing so. Be sure to breathe heavily, keep the elbows in, and hold the chest high.

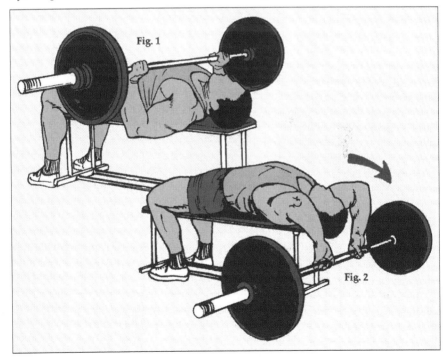

Fig. 1

Fig. 2

STANDING BARBELL TOE RAISE

Muscle Group: Main calf muscles
Degree of Difficulty: Intermediate

Place a barbell on the back of your shoulders. Step on a thick board or raised platform. Place your feet on the raised object to help balance yourself and to get a full extension and contraction of the calf muscle. Place your heels down. Inhale and push up on your toes as shown in illustration #1. This position is the flexed portion of the exercise and the lowering of the heels is the extension portion. Both are important. Do the exercise slowly and deliberately. Inhale as you raise on your toes and exhale as you lower your heels. If you turn your toes out and heels in, it will affect the inner calf more. If you keep your feet straight, it will affect the main calf muscle more. If you turn your toes in and heels out, it will affect the outside of the calf more.

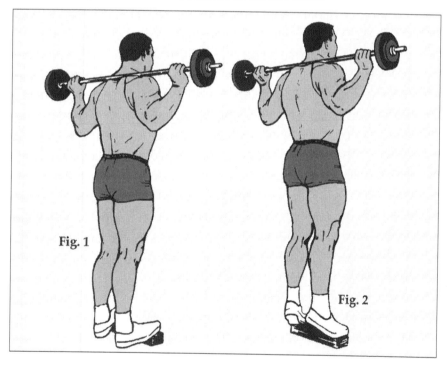

Fig. 1

Fig. 2

MEDIUM GRIP BARBELL UPRIGHT ROWING

Muscle Group: Front deltoids and trapezius
Degree of Difficulty: Intermediate

Place your hands on a barbell with the palms facing down and use a hand grip about eighteen inches apart. With the barbell at arm's length while you are standing erect and in a stationary position, pull the weight straight up until it is nearly under the chin. Keep the elbows out to the sides and in the top position the elbows are nearly as high as your ears. Keep the barbell in close to the body and pause momentarily at the top before letting the weight back to starting position. Inhale as you raise the bar and exhale as you lower the bar.

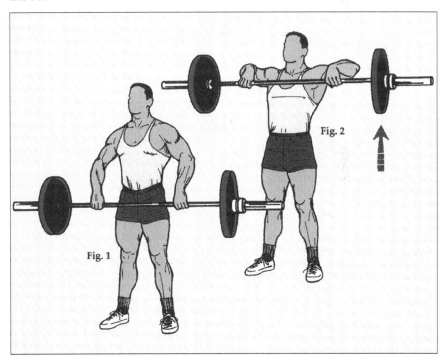

Fig. 1

Fig. 2

STANDING MILITARY PRESS

Muscle Group: Front and outer deltoids
Degree of Difficulty: Intermediate

This is the standard military press. Clean the weight to the chest. Lock the legs and hips solidly. This will give you a solid platform from which to push. Keep the elbows in slightly and under the bar, press the weight overhead, lock the arms out. When lowering the barbell to the upper chest, be sure it rests on the chest and is not held with the arms. If the chest is held high, it will give you a nice shelf on which to place the barbell and to push from. Inhale before the press and exhale when lowering the barbell.

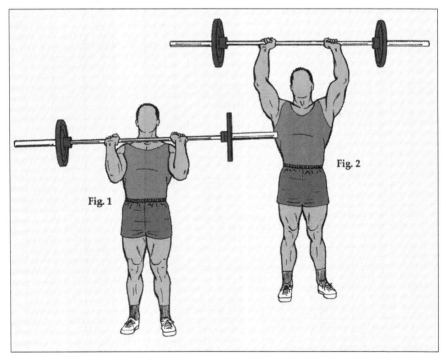

Fig. 1

Fig. 2

HAND ON BENCH ONE ARM DUMBBELL ROWING

Muscle Group: Upper and lower lats
Degree of Difficulty: Intermediate

Place a dumbbell on the floor in front of a bench. Put your left leg back, keeping your left knee locked. Bend the right leg slightly as you bend down and grasp the dumbbell with your left hand, using a palms in grip. Place your right hand on the bench and lock the elbow. With the dumbbell in your left hand hanging straight down and off the floor about six inches, inhale and pull the dumbbell straight up to the side of your chest, keeping your arm in close. Return to starting position and exhale. Do the prescribed number of repetitions on the right side and then change positions to the left side doing the same number of repetitions. Be sure the dumbbell does not touch the floor once the exercise has begun.

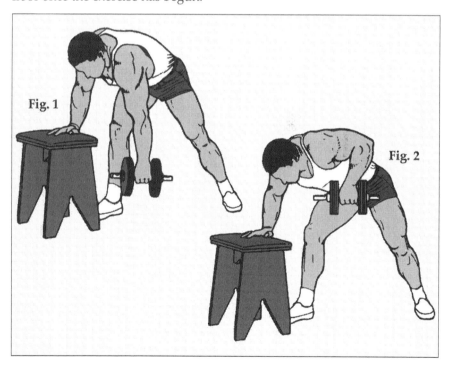

Fig. 1

Fig. 2

BARBELL DEAD LIFT

Muscle Group: Lower back

Degree of Difficulty: Intermediate

Place a barbell on the floor in front of you. With your feet about sixteen inches apart, bend down and grasp the bar just to the outside of your knees in the middle of your lower legs. Keep your knees bent and your back straight while you have your head up. Inhale and, using your thighs and back, stand erect with your arms locked out. Lower the weight to the floor and exhale.

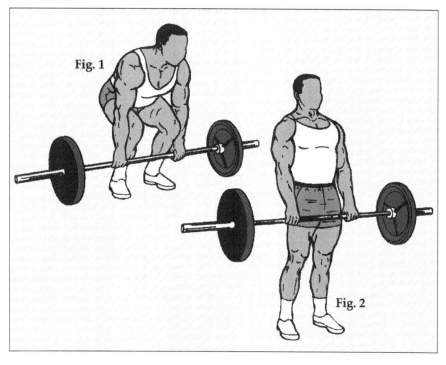

Fig. 1

Fig. 2

INCLINE LATERAL

Muscle Group: Upper pectorals
Degree of Difficulty: Intermediate

Use a hand position on the dumbbells similar to that of holding a barbell. Start with the dumbbells together at arm's length above the shoulders. Slowly lower them to the down position so the dumbbells are approximately even with the chest but about ten inches from each side of the chest. Notice that the elbows are drawn downwards and back so they are in line with the ears. The forearms are slightly out of a vertical position. The press back to starting position is done by using the same arc as in letting the dumbbells down. Inhale at the beginning of the exercise and exhale at the finish.

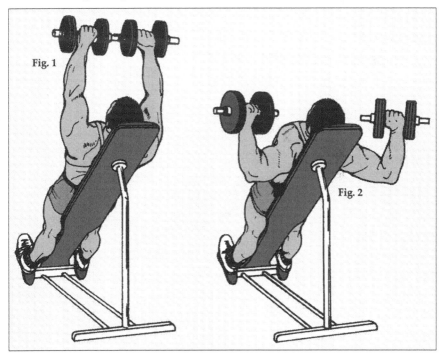

Fig. 1

Fig. 2

BENT ARM LATERAL

Muscle Group: Outer pectorals
Degree of Difficulty: Intermediate

Lie on a flat bench with the dumbbells together at arm's length above the shoulders The palms of the hands should be facing each other. Slowly lower the dumbbells to the down position so the dumbbells are approximately even with the chest but out about ten inches from each side of the chest. Notice that the elbows are drawn downwards and back so they are in line with the ears. The forearms are slightly out of a vertical position. The press back to starting position is done by using the same arc as in letting the dumbbells down. Inhale at the beginning of the exercise and exhale at the finish.

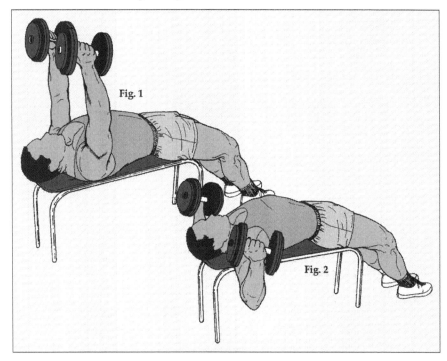

Fig. 1

Fig. 2

STANDING DUMBBELL TRICEPS CURL

Muscle Group: Triceps
Degree of Difficulty: Difficult

Grasp one dumbbell with both hands and raise it overhead to arm's length, vertical with the floor. As you are raising the dumbbell rotate your hands up and over until the top plates are resting in the palms of your hands while your thumbs remain around the handle. Stand erect with your back straight, head up and feet about sixteen inches apart. Keep your upper arms in close to the sides of your head during the exercise. Inhale and lower the dumbbell behind your head in a semicircular motion until your forearms and biceps touch. Return the weight to starting position using a similar path and exhale.

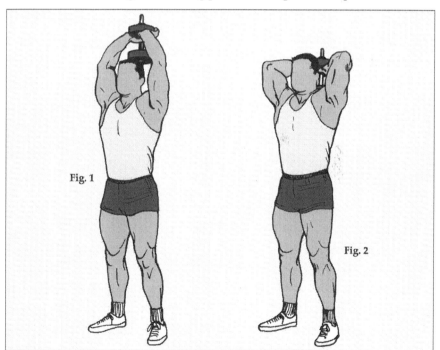

Fig. 1

Fig. 2

STANDING DUMBBELL CURL

Muscle Group: Biceps
Degree of Difficulty: Intermediate

Hold a dumbbell in each hand and stand erect with your feet about sixteen inches apart. Keep your back straight, head up, and hips and legs locked out. With the dumbbells hanging at arm's length at your sides, with your palms in, inhale and curl the dumbbells up to the height of your shoulders. As you commence the curl and the dumbbells are past your thighs, then turn your palms-up and keep them in this position throughout the exercise until you are lowering the weights and again near your upper thighs before turning your palms in again and exhaling. Keep your upper arms in close to your sides and concentrate on your biceps raising and lowering the weights.

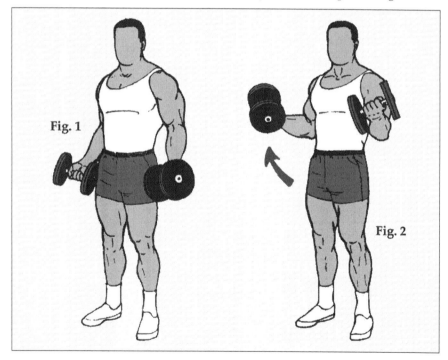

Fig. 1

Fig. 2

This page has been intentionally left blank.

Chapter 7

Course Three

EXERCISES:

1. Bent Knee Sit-Up	1 set of 25
2. Weighted Leg Raise	2 sets of 25
3. Medium Grip Incline Barbell Bench Press	5 sets of 5
4. Standing Palms in Alternated Dumbbell Press	5 sets of 5
5. Medium Grip Bent Over Barbell Rowing	3 sets of 6
6. Bent Arm Barbell Pullover	3 sets of 8
7. Standing Medium Grip Barbell Curl	4 sets of 6
8. Standing Close Grip Barbell Triceps Curl	4 sets of 6
9. Flat Footed Wide Stance Barbell Squat to Bench	5 sets of 5

- Follow this course of exercises for a six weeks period
- Do Three Workouts per Week

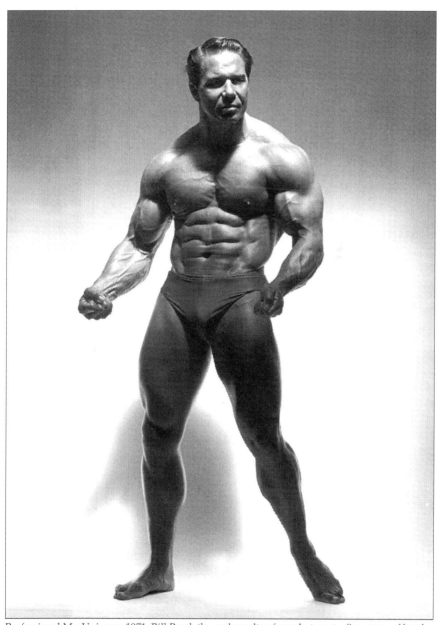

Professional Mr. Universe 1971. Bill Pearl, the end results of nearly twenty-five years of hard, continuous weight training.

BENT KNEE SIT-UP

Muscle Group: Upper abdominals
Degree of Difficulty: Intermediate

Sit down on a sit-up board and hook your feet under the strap. With your knees bent to about a 45° angle, put your hands behind your head and place your chin on your chest. This will keep a slight bow to your back. From this position, inhale and lie back until your lower back touches the board. Exhale as you return to starting position.

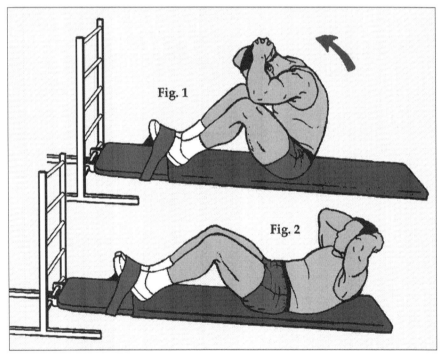

Fig. 1

Fig. 2

WEIGHTED LEG RAISE

Muscle Group: Lower abdominals
Degree of Difficulty: Difficult

Place a light dumbbell between your feet and lie supine on the floor with your hands under your buttocks, palms facing down. Keep your legs straight and your knees locked out. Inhale and raise your legs to a vertical position over your hips. Let your legs back to the floor and exhale.

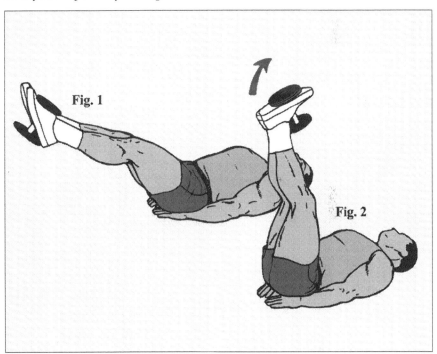

Fig. 1

Fig. 2

MEDIUM GRIP INCLINE BARBELL BENCH PRESS

Muscle Group: Upper pectorals
Degree of Difficulty: Intermediate

Lie back on an incline bench. Using a hand grip that is about six inches wider than your shoulder width, lower the barbell from arm's length above the shoulders to a position on the upper chest that is about three inches above the nipples of the pectorals. Note from the illustrations that the elbows are back. Inhale as you lower the weight to the upper chest and exhale as you press it back to arm's length above the shoulders. Do not relax and drop the weight to the upper chest but lower it in a controlled manner, making a definite pause at the upper chest before pressing it back to arm's length. Keep your head on the bench and hold your chest high but do not let the hips raise off the bench.

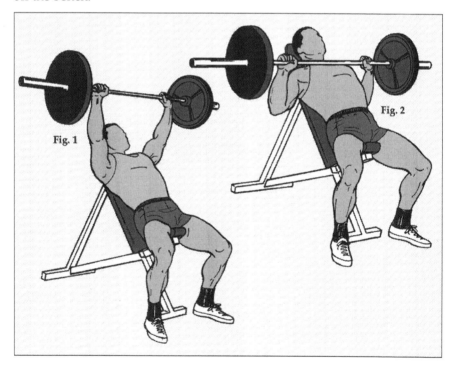

Fig. 1

Fig. 2

STANDING PALMS IN ALTERNATED DUMBBELL PRESS

Muscle Group: Front and outer deltoids
Degree of Difficulty: Intermediate

Clean two dumbbells to shoulder height. Lock the legs and hips solidly. Keep the elbows in slightly and have the palms of your hands facing each other. Take a deep breath and press the right arm straight up over your right shoulder. As you commence to lower the right arm, begin to press the left arm to arm's length above your left shoulder, letting the air out as the left arm is raised. Be sure to keep the palms of the hands facing each other during the entire exercise.

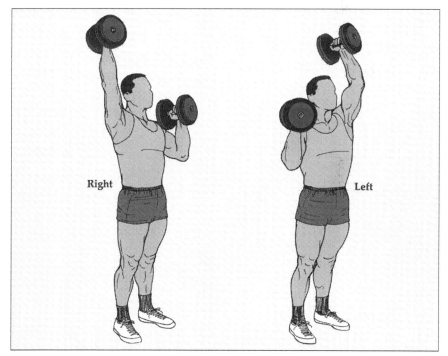

MEDIUM GRIP BENT OVER BARBELL ROWING

Muscle Group: Lats
Degree of Difficulty: Intermediate

Place a barbell on the floor in front of you. With your feet about eighteen inches apart bend down and get a grip on the barbell that is about twenty-six inches wide. Keep the legs bent and your back parallel to the floor as you inhale and pull the barbell directly up to the lower part of your chest. Exhale as the barbell returns to starting position. Do not let the barbell touch the floor once you have begun the exercise. Keep your head up and your back straight.

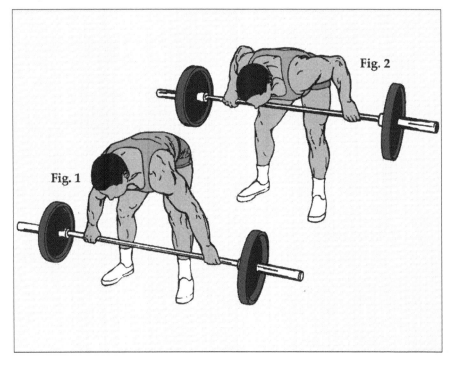

Fig. 2

Fig. 1

BENT ARM BARBELL PULLOVER

Muscle Group: Upper pectorals and rib cage
Degree of Difficulty: Intermediate

Lie supine on a flat bench with your shoulders at the end of the bench and your head pointing downward towards the floor. With a barbell on your chest resting in line with the nipples of the pectorals, use a hand grip that is about fourteen inches wide. Keeping the elbows in during the entire exercise, take a deep breath and lower the weight over your chest and face, keeping the barbell as close to the body as you can without scraping your nose. Continue to lower the weight until it touches the floor, or as low as is a comfortable position for you. Pull the barbell back to the chest, using the same path in which you lowered it. Exhale as you are doing so. Be sure to breathe heavily, keep the elbows in, and hold the chest high.

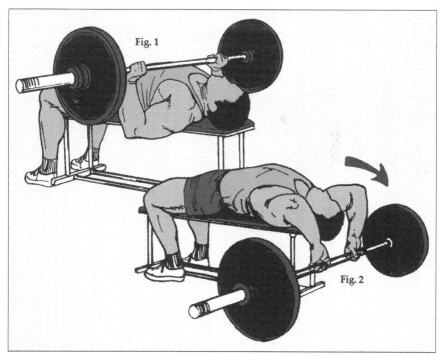

Fig. 1

Fig. 2

STANDING MEDIUM GRIP BARBELL CURL

Muscle Group: Biceps
Degree of Difficulty: Intermediate
Hold a barbell with both hands using a palms-up grip about eighteen inches apart. Stand erect with your feet about sixteen inches apart. With the barbell at arm's length against your upper thighs, inhale and curl the bar up to the height of your shoulders keeping your back straight, legs and hips locked out. As you are lowering the bar back to starting position, do so in a controlled manner causing the biceps to resist the weight as much as possible. Exhale as you return to starting position.

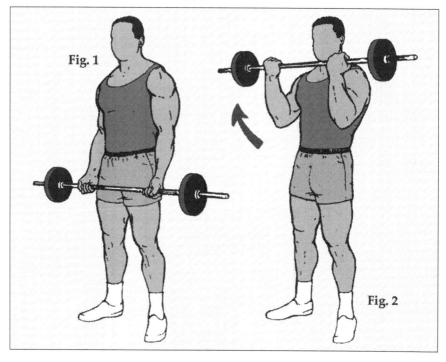

Fig. 1

Fig. 2

STANDING CLOSE GRIP BARBELL TRICEPS CURL

Muscle Group: Triceps
Degree of Difficulty: Intermediate

Hold a barbell with both hands using a palms down grip about six inches apart. Stand erect with your back straight, head up, hips and legs locked out. Press the barbell overhead to arm's length. Inhale and lower the weight straight down behind your head in a semicircular motion by bending your arms at the elbows but keeping your upper arms vertical throughout the exercise. The barbell should be lowered until your forearms and biceps touch. Press the barbell back to starting position using the same path and exhale. Be sure to keep your upper arms as close to the sides of your head as possible during the exercise.

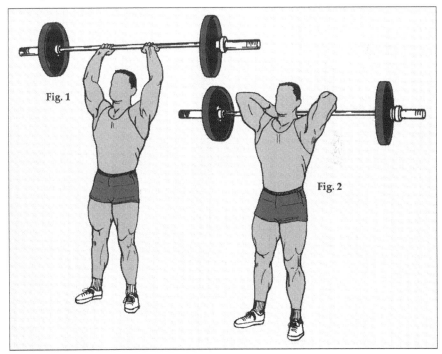

Fig. 1

Fig. 2

FLAT FOOTED WIDE STANCE BARBELL SQUAT TO BENCH

Muscle Group: Inner thighs
Degree of Difficulty: Intermediate

Place a bench that is about sixteen inches high behind you and stand close enough to the bench so your heels are about even with the end of the bench closest to you. Place a barbell on your upper back. Help stabilize the bar with a hand grip and spacing that feels most comfortable to you. Keep your head up, back straight, and your feet planted firmly on the floor about thirty inches apart. Inhale and squat down until your buttocks touch the bench. Do not take the tension off your thighs and totally sit on the bench. Your head should remain up, back straight, and your knees pointing outward. Return to starting position and exhale.

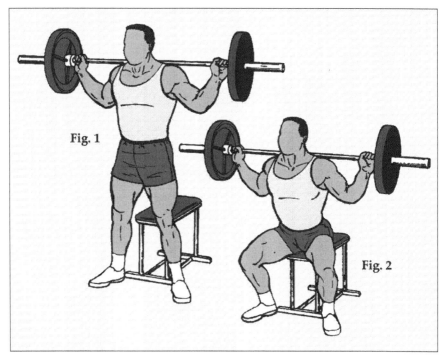

Fig. 1

Fig. 2

This page has been intentionally left blank.

Chapter 8

Diet

It is very difficult to recommend a diet for everyone using this book. Several things have to be considered. First, individual taste in foods; second, economic conditions; third, locale and availability of items suggested. Some persons are allergic to certain foods and cannot eat them under any circumstances. From a medical standpoint, one's doctor would not recommend such a diet. Therefore, we can only enlighten you about which foods are suitable and will produce the best results. You must choose the diet best suited for you. It is always a good idea to check with your family physician before starting ANY diet.

A person's environment and the attitude of the rest of the family about eating something entirely foreign to their normally prepared meals also has to be taken into consideration. We do not wish to recommend that a person follow a specific diet and cause conflict with the rest of the family. We feel it is best to recommend certain things and if they fit into your own particular situation, use them.

Starting your day with a good breakfast is very important. You will fortify your body with the fuel it needs to get the body operating efficiently. Protein is very important. Your body is largely made of protein. The muscles and internal organs require a supply of protein. Eat the foods that will give you the proper amount of protein. If possible, 50-75 grams, plus some fats and carbohydrates for balance.

Your lunch and dinner should be eaten at regular times, if possible. Eat a comfortable amount. If you find this is not enough to afford you the required amount of calories, start eating four to five times a day. You may also make outstanding gains by drinking a quart of milk during your workouts. If you do this, do not drink the milk cold. It is best to hold the cold liquid in your mouth until it is near body temperature before swallowing. When the stomach is over-heated through vigorous exercise, cramps will result when something cold is consumed.

According to reports, the average man consumes 2400-2800 calories a day. Bear in mind that this is average. It is not recommended that a person working out on a program such as we have outlined would be able to in-

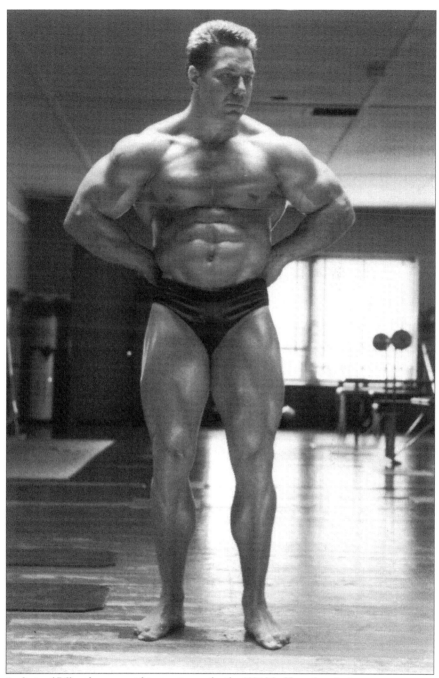

A photo of Bill, as he prepared to guest pose for the 1956 Mr. Hawaii contest.

crease body-weight and size on this amount. It is best to raise the caloric intake to about 5,000 a day, depending on the individual's assimilation and his age and size. Some persons require more calories than others. You will have to judge for yourself. This can be best determined by your progress after a short period of training.

Foods suitable for gaining bulk and power:

Vegetables, Soups, Grain Products

	Amount	Protein	Calories
Avocado	1/2 medium	2	263
Broccoli Stems	3/4 cup	2	35
Sprouts	3/4 cup	4	55
Barley (Whole)	1/2 cup	4	310
Corn (On Cob)	1 medium	3	90
Corn (Canned)	1/2 Cup	4	120
Hominy (White)	1/2 cup	0	355
Kidney Beans (Cooked)	1/2 cup	6	88
Lima Beans (Cooked)	1/2 cup	7	116
Navy Beans (Cooked)	1/2 cup	6	129
Peas (Fresh)	1/2 cup	7	100
Potatoes (Baked)	1 medium	3	92
Potatoes (Sweet)	1 medium	3	130
Yams	1 medium	2	150
Rice, Brown (Cooked)	3/4 cup	4	117
Rice, Polished (Cooked)	3/4 cup	2	117
Soya Beans, Dry (Uncooked)	3/4 cup	51	270
Soya Beans (Cooked)	1/2 cup	20	108
String Beans	3/4 cup	2	43
Cream of Tomato Soup	3/4 cup	4	143
Spaghetti	3/4 cup	3	127
Macaroni (White, Cooked)	3/4 cup	3	130
Corn Flakes	3/4 cup	2	100
Oatmeal (Cooked)	1/2 cup	4	80
Shredded Wheat	1 Biscuit	3	108
Corn Meal (White)	1/2 cup	8	270
Buckwheat Flour	1 cup	6	387

	Amount	Protein	Calories
Rye Bread	1 slice	3	76
Wheat Germ	1/2 cup	24	220
Whole Wheat Bread (100%)	1 slice	3	75
Graham Crackers	2	2	84

Meats

	Amount	Protein	Calories
Bacon (Crisp)	1 1/2 slices	2	53
Beef (Lean)	1 slice	22	190
Bologna	10 small slices	8	109
Beef Brains	4 oz	11	127
Chicken	4 oz	18	125
Corned Beef	4 oz	16	196
Frankfurters	2 links	14	224
Ham	4 oz	20	248
Heart (Beef)	4 oz	17	96
Lamb Chops	2 chops	20	359
Lamb Roasted	4 oz	22	225
Lentils (Cooked)	1/2 cup	9	115
Liver (Beef)	4 oz, 1 slice	20	140
Liver (Calf)	4 oz, 1 slice	23	148
Liver (Chicken)	4 oz	20	130
Mutton Leg	4 oz	20	191
Pork Chops	2 chops	14	340
Pork Sausage	6 links	10	402
Rabbit	4 oz	20	192
Steak (Beef)	1 slice	21	156
Tongue (Beef)	1 slice	16	226
Turkey	4 oz	24	153
Veal Cutlets	4 oz	20	184
Veal Chops	2 chops	19	209

Fish

	Amount	Protein	Calories
Fish	avg. serving	21	140
Herring	4 oz	19	394

Salmon	4 oz	22	203
Sardines, Canned	4 oz	13	103
Tuna, Canned	1/4 cup	9	64
Cod Fish	4 oz	16	70
Cod Fish Oil	1 tablespoon	0	100

Milk & Cheeses

	Amount	Protein	Calories
American Cheese	2"x1"x1" piece	12	160
Cheddar Cheese	2 tablespoons	7	100
Cottage Cheese	1/2 cup	20	100
Swiss Cheese	1 slice	10	135
Fresh Whole Milk	1 quart	33	660
Fresh Skimmed Milk	1 quart	34	370
Dried Skim Milk	1/2 cup	35	350
Buttermilk	1 quart	30	400
Goat's Milk	1 quart	32	672
Condensed Milk	1/2 cup	9	326
Whole Egg	1	6	75
Egg Yolk	1	3	58

Dressings & Spreads

	Amount	Protein	Calories
Butter	1 square	0	77
Corn Oil	1 tablespoon	0	100
Olive Oil	1 tablespoon	0	135
Honey	1 tablespoon	0	101
Margarine	1 oz	0	261
Mayonnaise	1 tablespoon	0	100
Peanut Butter	2 tablespoons	0	203

Pastries & Desserts

	Amount	Protein	Calories
Custard	1/2 cup	7	126
Chocolate Pudding	1/2 cup	5	272
Tapioca (Cooked)	1/2 cup	0	118

Doughnuts	2	7	481
Cookies, Molasses	1 large	2	100
Ice Cream	1/2 cup	2	208
Chocolate Malted Milk	13 oz	11	514
Chocolate Milk Shake	13 oz	10	472
Chocolate Candy with Nuts	1 bar	5	219
Milk Chocolate Candy	1 bar	4	282

Fruits & Nuts

	Amount	Protein	Calories
Almonds	10 medium	2	65
Apple	1 small	0	64
Applesauce	1/2 cup	1	42
Apricots	4 dried	1	102
Apricots (Fresh)	6 halves	1	70
Banana	1 medium	1	85
Cashews	20 Nuts	6	202
Cranberry Sauce	3/4 cup	0	300
Dates (Dried)	15 medium	2	347
Figs (Dried)	2 small	1	103
Figs (Fresh)	2 large	1	42
Orange Juice (Fresh)	1 cup	1	110
Peanuts	18 Nuts	5	110
Pecans	10 large	3	229
Walnuts (English)	1/2 cup	5	197
Prunes (Dried)	6 medium	2	173
Raisins (Seeded)	1/2 cup	1	105

Some of the most concentrated yet inexpensive proteins are:
- Brewers Yeast
- Wheat Germ
- Soy Flour
- Dry Milk

It is best to consume the amount of Calories and Protein in relation to your age and size. A good book to purchase should you wish to really go into the subject of diet is *Lets Eat Right to Keep Fit* by Adelie Davis.

Chapter 9

Training Notes

Work in Relation to Training

Many men, who work in a physical capacity each day, become discouraged when training with weights. Their feeling is that at the end of a hard day's labor, their energy is depleted, and they are incapable of a thorough workout with weights. Many "white collar" workers are taxed with mental fatigue, which, actually, creates a real physical fatigue.

Whichever category you fail within, be realistic and work within your capabilities. Proper diet is essential when working (be it physical or mental) and training. You must consume enough food to handle your normal duties and training, plus a little more to build a reserve. If you are not making the normal gains, you must adjust your training program and find which is the right amount of work to produce the best results. To make gains in training, one has to train hard, but be aware of the danger of over-training.

In case of an injury, it is wise to substitute an exercise that will not irritate the injury, or eliminate the exercise altogether until you have fully recovered. I you should have a bad back, give special attention to warming up. Never, under any circumstances, round your back when squatting or executing the dead lifts. Remover that your body gives warning. Don't push yourself beyond your limitations.

Strength in Relation to Size

Many people argue that one becomes stronger if he increases his bodyweight. In most cases this is not true. Usually, a person gains only fat, and this is more detrimental than valuable.

You should strive to gain the right kind of bodyweight. This can be accomplished by correct training, heavy weights, proper foods, and plenty of rest and relaxation. Remember, consistency in your training and good daily habits are of prime importance.

Training Hints

Several important rules should be taken into consideration when em-

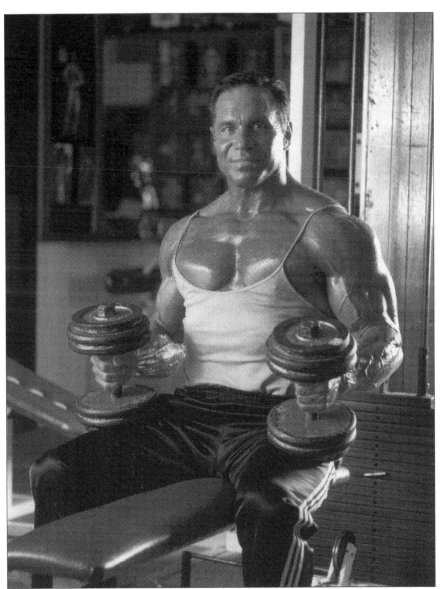

This photo was taken on Bill's 55th birthday just prior to his giving a posing exhibition at the Derby Invitational physique contest in Derby, England. Photograph by Chris Lund.

barking on a Bulk and Power Program. Be regular in your eating and sleeping habits; follow a well-planned program; have the proper mental attitude towards training and everyday living. If any of these rules are broken, the end results may not be as rewarding as desired.

It is our hope to get you started properly in these important areas in order to save you hundreds of wasted hours of "trial and error" to obtain the same principles we have discovered in our years of training champions in all fields of athletics and bodybuilding.

A diet of good wholesome food, properly prepared and taken at the same time each day, will product better results than irregular eating habits and haphazard planning of meals.

Sleep and relaxation are also important and should not be overlooked in building bulk and power. Because everyone has a different physical make-up, one cannot say that an exact amount of sleep will be proper for all persons. However, we feel that eight hours sleep per night should be sufficient. Ten hours sleep a night should be considered maximum. Going to bed at the same time every night is very effective and helps the system to regulate itself and produce a faster increase in bodyweight. The ability to relax is a great asset to anyone seeking added bodyweight and strength.

A proper mental attitude plays a large role in your efforts to build size and strength. When thinking positive thoughts, one has a happy outlook on life. You should think positively about all your daily activities, physical, mental, and moral. It will aid you in your training in the gym, as well as your personal life. A healthy, positive attitude will improve your body and help make you a better person.

83586478R00038

Made in the USA
San Bernardino, CA
27 July 2018